© by Juan Antonio de Blas de Miguel, 2021
© Cover and illustrations by Rosa Álvarez Halcón
© Video by José Daniel Sanz
© Translation by Elena Margioli

Neither the author nor the publisher are responsible for any improper use of the training techniques and methods described in the present publication.
First edition published 2021.

More info (in Spanish)
www.centrodantian.com

TAI CHI
FOR OLDER PEOPLE
A method to improve health

Juan Antonio de Blas

Aknowledgements:

To my Sifu, Pedro Rico
To Rosa Álvarez Halcón, for the Art
To J. Daniel Sanz, for the video edition
To Ana Labarías, for the photographs
To Paco Godina, for the technical advice

...and an honorable mention to my grandmother, Margarita Lahoz, for reaching the age of 100 without knowing anything about Tai Chi.

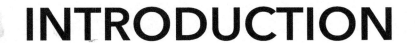

INTRODUCTION

"Knowing others is wisdom.
Knowing yourself is enlightenment.
He who conquers others is strong; he
who conquers himself is mighty."

This book was born with the aim of being a practical and simple manual that will constitute a useful tool for older people who wish to maintain or increase their general state of health. Throughout my teaching experience with this group, I have been able to observe how the application of the basic principles and traditional Tai Chi training methods make up an ideal work system in this sense and an instrument for constant growth and improvement. Thus, the content of this book arises from my experience working specifically with older people for fifteen years.

Without a doubt, most of the issues that are tackled here could be analysed more profoundly. However, this increase in the level of proximity to the theory and training of Tai Chi Chuan would be detrimental to the initial purpose of the book. In consequence, I will try to maintain a reasonable balance between richness and specificity, so that the text is manageable and practical, without losing the didactic quality befitting a publication of these characteristics.

WHAT IS
TAI CHI?

"All know the way, but few actually walk it."

APPEARANCE AND ESSENCE: WHAT IS TAI CHI?

The importation of all kinds of oriental disciplines, to the United States, at first, and later to Europe, since the decades of the sixties and the seventies, has given rise to a long series of mistakes and misunderstandings. In the particular case of Tai Chi, the traditional systems have become, too often, a kind of "soft gymnastics", or "meditation in motion", originated by the necessity to pack up and distribute this discipline as a consumable product from which to get the highest possible credit. Additionally, and because the majority of the public interested in getting to know these disciplines lacked previous information, not a few have been those who have tried to pontificate from an unqualified position, founded on incomplete learning methods, far removed from the high standards of the traditional teaching under the tutelage of Masters associated with the original lineages.

Fortunately, this detrimental tendency has been experiencing a process of reversion for some years now. This is thanks to the qualified and respectable work of many traditional Masters who, with their schools and publications, have taken it upon themselves to keep the essence of this Chinese Art alive. In addition, it's becoming more and more frequent to see technical texts published, as well as didactic material presented in various media, which offer accurate, confirmed information on these matters. Their transmission and systematization have been based on the oral tradition for countless generations of Sifus (Masters).

Tai Chi Chuan is, and always has been, a Martial Art; that is to say, a fighting system. It is a Martial Art, and nothing else.

I think it's extremely important to stress this since, although in this book I am not going to delve into the martial aspects of Tai Chi, it is necessary to know what things are and what they are not in order not to, even despite using them outside their context to develop specific objectives, deviate from their essence nor adulterate them.

In this sense, it is the teachers' obligation to preserve the tradition of Tai Chi as pure as possible and transmit it without diluting it or contaminating it.

Furthermore, and beyond the context of the dissemination and conservation of the traditional styles of Tai Chi Chuan, their systematic study and training offer a series of benefits for the practitioner, some of which I will go on to enumerate in the next section.

THE BENEFITS OF TAI CHI

Older people present, in general, a series of characteristics that must be taken into consideration when undertaking proper work of conditioning and improvement. The very nature of Tai Chi Chuan offers us a wide range of resources to initiate an excellent training program. On the whole, we can divide the benefits that we will obtain from our practice into two big categories: internal and external benefits.

- Internal benefits:

In Martial Arts, internal work is understood as everything related to the management of the Energy, or *Chi*, of our body. We are not going to delve into these questions, as they are complex matters that deserve a more extensive analysis. However, we will understand as internal work that which has to do with our breathing, the relaxation of our Mind and Spirit (*Shen*), and the enhancement of the natural circulation of Chi when we perform the exercises. In the martial context of Tai Chi, this state of harmony has the purpose of increasing the efficiency of the techniques, by eliminating any type of physical tension and allowing us to control Chi.

- External benefits:

In contrast to internal work, external work is aimed, from a martial point of view, at physical conditioning and strengthening. These improvements are not an end in and of themselves, but a consequence of training. The most relevant ones are muscle tone increase, strengthening and elasticizing the connective tissue, and increasing bone density. It should be noted that all these factors directly depend on the intensity and frequency of our training.

In addition to all this, the work in Tai Chi Chuan offers another series of very beneficial factors for older people. Knee and leg muscle strengthening translates into balance improvement, which reduces the probability of suffering a fall. Other faculties are also developed, such as coordination and the ability to concentrate. We will talk about all this more extensively in later sections.

Before ending this chapter, I would like to stress that the student's goal should be to contribute, through the training systems that will be described further down, to improving their general state of health, always in the context of a healthy lifestyle and combined with other elements of equal importance in this respect. In no case is it reasonable to place blind faith in any discipline. Nor, of course, can it replace any treatment prescribed by a medical practitioner.

BRIEF HISTORY OF TAI CHI CHUAN

As I have indicated in the introduction, this book seeks to be a simple and accessible manual; for this reason, I will not narrate a History of Tai Chi Chuan truffled with names, dates and historical facts. This would unnecessarily thicken the text and would make it less accessible and manageable. However, it is advisable to get to know some aspects, people and events that make up the soul of our Art, so that you can take in certain facets of the daily work in Tai Chi.

Tai Chi is one of the oldest Martial Arts in existence and, though it would be difficult to determine exactly when it originated as such, the first existing documents date back to approximately fifteen hundred years ago. The *Tai Chi Chuan* syntagm can be translated to English as *supreme boxing*; such was the trust that the ancient Masters put in this fighting system.

At first, the different styles of Tai Chi Chuan that we know today didn't exist. They started to appear as the Sifus of different lineages started to develop their own methods and viewpoints around the techniques. For this reason, the numerous Tai Chi styles that are practised today worldwide receive the name of the distinct lineages that gave them shape. In my case, I am part of the lineage of the Yang family, the most widespread Tai Chi style, whose principles and methods we are going to study in this book. However, it is useful to remember that, as I've already mentioned, there are multiple Tai Chi styles. They are all worthy of the same respect by any serious Martial Arts practitioner. The most widespread systems are Yang, Chen, Wu, Hao and Sun.

The texts from which we can get part of Tai Chi history are scarce, and their discovery is relatively recent. Most of the data come from the oral tradition; for which reason, many facts might have been adulterated or made up during the successive transmissions of the information. It is therefore complicated to situate certain events with certainty and precisely pinpoint every agent who participated in the creation and development of Tai Chi.

As the tradition of our lineage recounts, one of the first Masters to reach certain notoriety among his community was Xu Xin-Ping, a disciple of Master Yu Huan-Zi, from whom he learned the 37 techniques of Tai Chi, very similar to some of the most important ones among the techniques that we have today. Master Xu became famous for his quaint personality, as well as for his wisdom and ability in combat. It was said that he lived secluded in the mountains, and he went down to the civilization to sell firewood and buy wine. Master Xu was said to be tall and very strong, with a long, white beard and, under his robe, a body forged by the harshness of martial training. He was bright-eyed and "able to run like a horse." The songs and legends around his figure are numerous. This Master lived during the Tang period and is considered by many scholars one of the first Masters to have helped Tai Chi be introduced, little by little, to the culture of the Chinese people.

Later in time, the traces of the first verified documents take us to the figure of the erudite Zhang San-Feng (XIII century). Sifu Zhang was a high official of the Chinese government, who, halfway through his life, decided to retire to Mount Hua to meditate and carry out his studies. Later, his pilgrimage took him to the famous mountain of Wu Dang, in the province of Hubei, to delve into the precepts of Taoism. At that time of his life, Master Zhang was about seventy years old and dedicated himself to tutoring Taoist monks in Tai Chi to keep fit, at the same time as studying their famous methods of Chi Kung to achieve longevity. During this phase of his studies, he came to the conclusion that it was necessary to perfect the internal facet of the combat in order to preserve the efficacy of the techniques during old age. Thus, he enunciated the four fundamental principles of classic Tai Chi Chuan:

- Soft against hard.
- Calm against action.
- Slow against fast.
- One against many.

These four principles should not be interpreted in a literal way, since they enclose a lot more complex concepts which exceed the aspirations of this manual. These are, roughly, the origins of Tai Chi Chuan. However, the principles of Tai Chi that we know today were established many generations later, by Chen Chang-Xing. This Master developed the first modern style of Tai Chi: The Ancient Chen, or Original Chen.

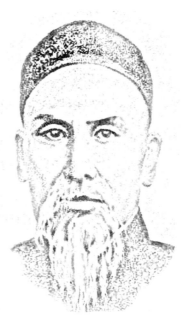

The founder of our style, Yang Lu-Chan, (1799-1872) became a disciple of Sifu Chen because he wanted to become stronger, and mainly to combat the severe chronic stomach ailments that he suffered from. Years later, Master Yang became known under the nickname *The Invincible*.

Yang Lu-Chan

Yang Lu-Chan had two sons: Yang Ban-Hon and Yang Jian-Hon, who carried on his work. However, it was the sons of Yang Jian-Hon who achieved the greatest popularity and played a vital role in the diffusion of Yang Tai Chi Chuan. These Masters were Yang Shou-Hou and Yang Cheng-Fu. It was the latter who carried out the most academic part of the work, since his brother Shou-Hou was characterized by a

18

high level of exigency and rudeness at the time of training his disciples, attitudes that alienated him from the vast majority. On the other hand, Master Yang Cheng-Fu became very famous and developed a great part of the technical work that has survived to this day. One of the fathers of our lineage studied under his tutelage: Grandmaster Hu Yuen-Chou. This great Master and doctor is remembered with respect and affection by the community of Tai Chi Chuan and Kung Fu practitioners, thanks to his great erudition and martial capacity. His work of education and dissemination opened the doors to several generations of Masters around the world, situating the original tradition of Yang outside the Chinese borders, by the hand of Sifu Doc-Fai Wong, who currently resides and teaches in the city of San Francisco. All of this is but a brief summary of the lengthy history of Tai Chi Chuan. Even though I could digress much more in the narration, I think that what has been written gives an accurate overall view for the reader to get a good idea of the remote origins of our Martial Art.

TECHNICAL
ASPECTS

"There are two ways of spreading light: to be the candle or the mirror that reflects it."

It is essential to carefully observe the theoretical and technical principles of any Martial Art in order to advance with guarantees of success in its learning. Despite the simplicity of the training and exercise systems proposed in this manual, there are some basic pillars that you have to know to perfection to start working productively, avoiding injuries and getting the greatest possible benefit out of daily practice.

Reaching technical perfection is the ideal of every martial artist. And even though it is frequent, at least for the inexperienced eye, to neglect this aspect in favour of the sensations that one can get to experience during practice, it is not acceptable to put aside the search for perfection and harmony in each of the learning phases.

There is broad agreement around the fact that the most important thing from a technical point of view in any martial system is stance. So that, if our stance is good, we can build an effective working method. It is so much so, that in many martial styles, the initial phases of training consist of the comprehension and development of correct postural work and footwork patterns.

In the case of Tai Chi, just like in many Kung Fu styles, this work can take months, consuming almost the totality of the training hours.

This idea can be daunting at first, since dedicating so much time and effort to this kind of work is not as gratifying as other parts of the study. Nevertheless, you must understand stance as the foundation on top of which to build all progress in your growth within the sphere of Tai Chi Chuan.

For this reason, before going any further, I am going to explain the how and the why of the basic stance of Tai Chi Yang, and how to perform a correct footwork.

THE BOW STANCE

The bow stance is the basis of the technique of Tai Chi Chuan Yang. For the reader to be able to comprehend and assimilate the reason for being of said stance, I will first explain three of the most important principles that set the basis for all our work:

The origin of power

Beyond the mere conditioning of the body for martial practice, the transmission of power to the push or impact point results from the sum of forces that act from the bottom up, and are effectively transmitted through the geometrically correct stance. One of the keys to the refinement of Tai Chi Chuan is, precisely, the perfection of its stances. So that, in the maximum state of relaxation possible, the martial artist is capable of producing great power without losing their centre; remaining anchored, or rooted, in the specific point where they execute the technique.

Turning the waist

Within the martial approach of Tai Chi (and of most traditional Chinese Martial Arts), it is understood that the whole body is the tool that punches, pushes or executes a lever joint locks or dislocation. Thus, it is not the fist that punches, but rather the whole body which transmits its power to the fist.

The waist takes on a key role in this process, adding power to the techniques. But, on top of that, the rotation of the waist produces what is colloquially called internal massage of the organs. We will delve into this matter in a bit.

Balance

It is obvious that no martial technique can be considered effective if it is executed in imbalance. This is one of the most important aspects of Tai Chi practice. The adequate management of the body weight becomes key to educate our balance and optimize our learning in Tai Chi.

Having in mind all that I have just explained, we are in a position to offer a detailed description of the bow stance. To take up a correct bow stance, we should take into account the following precepts:

The stance predisposes the movement, whether to execute a complete technique from the guard stance or to perform a step forward (we will talk about steps backward in due course). Taking this into account, the foot that is in front after performing a determined technique, and before moving, indicates the direction of the movement, while the back foot forms with it an angle of forty-five degrees.

This is so because forty-five degrees is the most our waist can rotate before tension is produced. For this reason, to obtain the greatest physical relaxation possible and improve our balance, we trace this angle with our feet.

The support points of our body must be separated to increase balance when performing the movements and techniques. We spread our feet breadthwise the distance determined by the two vertices of our waist rotation angle, and which equals, approximately, the width of our hips, a little more than the width of our shoulders. This opening is called the *third line* and it constitutes a fundamental aspect when building correct stance.

We should keep both knees bent at all times, trying not to elevate our position during the transitions from one technique to the next.

The back should remain straight, and the shoulders and rib cage relaxed.

It is necessary to tuck the pelvis to correct the curve of the spine in the lumbar region, and thus direct the weight of the torso to the soles of our feet. In a way, it could be said that in performing this simple gesture, we are "sitting standing."

The length between our feet should be sufficient for the knee in front to be parallel to the centre of the sole.

Now that we have seen the defining characteristics of the bow stance, you should practise it carefully until clearly assimilating all the constituent elements. At the same time, we will begin to work on moving forward, having in mind a fundamental principle: in order to always keep balance, most of the body weight must be on the limb that does not move. This way, every time we move a foot or a leg, this is free of weight. In Tai Chi we call *full leg*, or *Yang*, the leg that supports the weight of our body; while the leg that is free of weight, *Yin*, is *empty*. These same criteria are applied to the steps backwards likewise.

To establish a solid study base and advance more quickly to the assimilation of the diverse techniques that we will see in this manual, it is essential that you fully internalize this stance and steps work, since it constitutes the very foundation of Tai Chi Chuan.

Front view   *Side view*

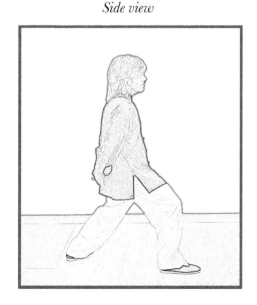

As an exercise, you should perform short sequences of steps forward and backward until dominating their mechanism. Being that, upon retreating, the weight of the body rests on the back leg, I recommend doing a smaller number of repetitions to avoid muscle overload and pain in the knees. Once this essential work is internalized, we can apply this basis to the training of complete Tai Chi techniques. This method of training is the most traditional way of learning.

MAXIMUM RELAXATION

Tai Chi Chuan is an Internal Martial Art. This means that in training one seeks to obtain the highest efficiency of a given technique through a strong and constant flow of Energy and not simply by strengthening the body. This is why it is said that a Tai Chi Master develops more martial power the older he gets, since he has managed to refine his Art over the years, and consciously and efficiently controls his internal Energy.

Although this remark about internal Martial Arts presents their reality from an excessively simplified point of view, it can orient you in the idea that, despite what many people may think at first, the more intense the relaxation, the greater the strength. This principle is of great importance, since the direct benefit that we can obtain from our daily practice largely depends on it. Despite not being interested in the martial application of our work, we must carefully take note of all these principles to maximize our benefit from it.

Hence, in our study, we should always seek maximum physical relaxation. To achieve it, we have to pay close attention to some important guidelines:

The back should always be as straight as possible. The whole spine should form, in a relaxed way, a straight line. To achieve this, it is important to try to tuck the pelvis in each of the positions, as if we were "seated". This simple move, apart from straightening the lumbar curve of the spine, also fulfils the purpose of directing all of our weight towards the soles of our feet, which relieves the load from the lumbar region and contributes to achieving rooting the position, an essential element of Tai Chi Chuan.

The shoulders should always be relaxed. Many people think, erroneously, that when they tense the trapezius muscle, they contribute to straightening the spine. Not only is this not the case, but putting the shoulders under unnecessary tension, something that is very common, impedes the correct transmission of the Energy, and often leads to contractures and problems caused by them, some of which are serious.

In Tai Chi, we never stretch the joints completely. The excessive tension of any joint makes the circulation of the Energy difficult, and it often goes hand-in-hand with the generation of stress in other joints. For this reason, you should seek balance in the extension of the limbs when executing the techniques and exercises.

The rib cage should also remain totally relaxed. In the same way as with the shoulders, some people associate the tension in the chest with a straight spine. This is not true. What is more, if there is tension in our chest, we are probably also putting tension in our shoulders, and, apart from that, abdominal breathing is rendered impossible.

BREATHING

This matter can be extremely complex, and it requires a much more extensive and in-depth analysis than the one foreseen for a manual of these characteristics. Adjusting to the purpose of this book, I am going to establish some general guidelines that we can apply to our daily training. Unlike most styles and lineages of Chi Kung, in the case of Tai Chi, it is not necessary to consciously control nor regulate breathing. When the traditional Masters were asked about this issue, they used to respond: "Do you control your breathing when you walk?" From this answer, we can deduce that we are looking for natural, relaxed breathing, which is automatically regulated as we perform the different techniques and Forms. We can also conclude that, the deeper the breathing, the slower will be, in turn, the speed at which the work is executed.

Obviously, this principle does not apply in a strict sense when one is looking to advance in Tai Chi from a martial perspective. But this is not something that we are going to deal with in this book. As a starting point, we will work with the idea of practising using soft, relaxed and constant breathing. We breathe air in and out always through the nose, avoiding doing so through the mouth. We breathe regularly and continuously, never retaining air nor breathing in to the point of reaching the maximum capacity of our lungs. In spite of how easy these guidelines are to understand, you should pay close attention to them and dedicate as much time as necessary to assimilate them correctly since, even if we understand everything perfectly, we may have to educate our body in this new attitude towards breathing. For someone who has been breathing in a certain way for all their lives, it is not easy to adopt new habits.

Once we have comprehended and assimilated all of this, we should highlight that it is always advisable to use abdominal breathing. This question should be presented and analysed in greater depth, and for this reason, it is excluded from this manual.

ZHANG ZHUANG: Traditional meditation

It is very relevant within the study of Tai Chi Chuan to see some meditative work and learn certain Chi Kung techniques that help students efficiently and consciously feel and regulate their Energy. It goes without saying that this part of the study can be extremely complicated and must be rigorously approached. Without a doubt, it would be necessary to write another book to treat this matter from a more thorough perspective. However, and far from such intention, I think it is appropriate to present two simple exercises that will help you achieve a greater degree of softness in your breathing, linking it to physical relaxation.

Doing these two exercises as preparation before practising Tai Chi will help you reach higher levels of physical relaxation and will prepare your mind to face the work from a more conscious standpoint.

Wu Chi (the ultimate nothingness)

The first step consists in adopting a correct stance to perform the exercise: feet are open to the width of the shoulders, the spine is straight, and the shoulders and chest are completely relaxed. Our hands should be placed at the sides, with our fingers spread and relaxed. The middle finger rests on the line outlined by the femur. If you wish, you can close your eyes to concentrate on the exercise more easily.

Once this stance has been adopted, it is necessary to regulate breathing. You should start breathing in the most relaxed way possible, trying to make the inspiration and the expiration of air last the same, without pausing between the two and without forcing lung capacity. You should feel your breathing soft and deep throughout the exercise. When you feel comfortable breathing with this method, it is the moment to advance to the next step: every time you exhale air, set your intention on gradually relaxing your shoulders more and more. Even though it seems like they're already relaxed, you will discover that with every breath you can reach a greater level of relaxation.

It is not advisable to perform this type of exercise for too long, especially at the early stages of training. A practice of five minutes suffices. Also, we should avoid forcing our breath or trying to continue if we feel any type of discomfort or uneasiness during the practice. It is better to stop and come back in another moment.

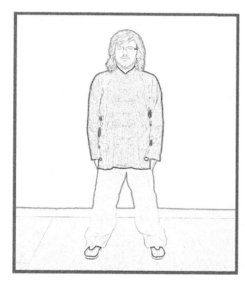 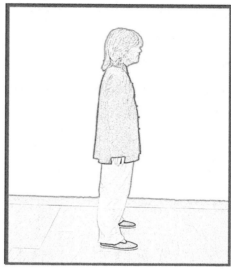

Front Vew   *Side view*

Fen Yuan (parting the clouds)

Through this exercise, you will learn to maintain soft and constant breathing while performing a dynamic practice in a state of relaxation.

The first step consists in taking up the bow stance, with your right leg forward. In this position, you should first shift the body weight to the left leg, placing both hands with the palms facing each other at the height of the navel without them touching. Next, and at the same time as distributing the weight between both legs, raise your arms in front of you until the elbows are almost extended. Then, turning your palms outwards, make a circle with your arms all the way to the initial position. While performing this exercise, you should maintain a relaxed gaze directed to the front, and without focusing on anything specific.

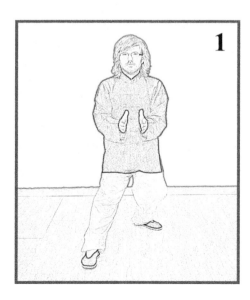
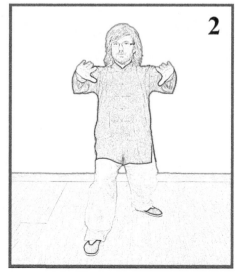

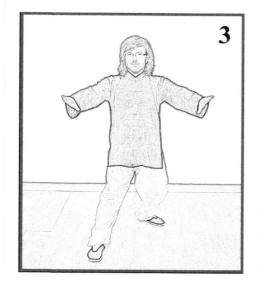
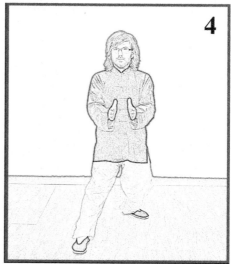

FIRST
STEPS

"The tree which fills the arms grew from the tiniest sprout; A journey of a thousand miles begins with a single step."

WARMING UP

Before starting any physical activity, whether it is light or more intense, it is indispensable that you do a full warm-up stretching, adequate to the activity you will undertake. Otherwise, you may get hurt or feel discomfort. Next, I describe a very simple table of exercises, which you can perform as preparation for any physical work. The number of repetitions and the duration of each exercise are suggestive and can be modified to fit each case. Of course, having in mind your state of health, you should eliminate from the table the exercises that could be detrimental to you or cannot be performed for whatever reason.

Gently move your head up and down, twelve times.

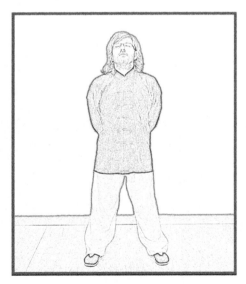 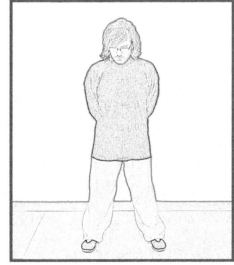

Rotate your neck from left to right, twelve times.

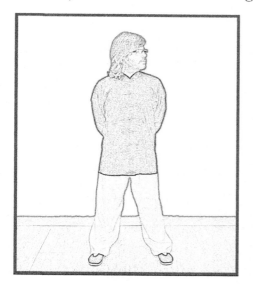 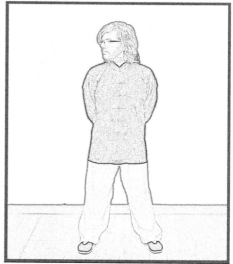

Move your head from shoulder to shoulder, twelve times.

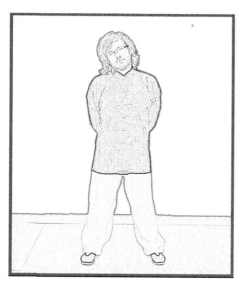 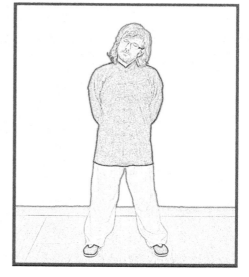

Rotate your head to one side and then to the other, twelve times in each direction. To avoid discomfort in the cervical area or dizziness, it is advisable not to force the movement during the part of the exercise in which the head is tilted backwards.

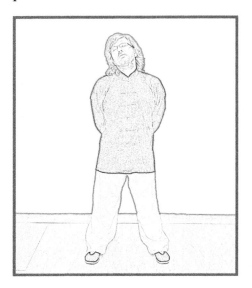 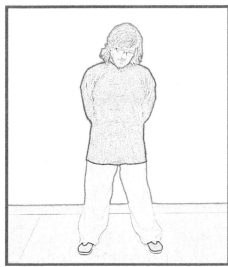

Rotate your shoulders, clockwise and counter-clockwise, twelve times in each direction.

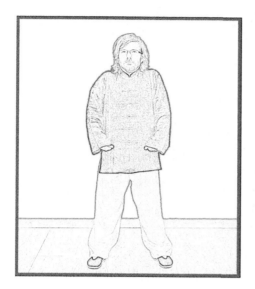 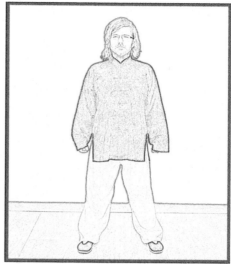

Placing one arm behind your head, and holding the elbow, gently stretch inwards for fifteen seconds. Repeat with the other arm.

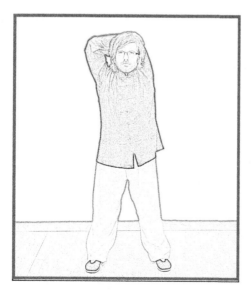 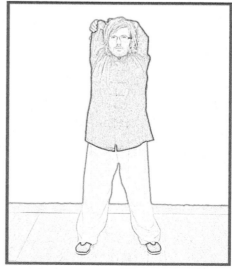

Placing one arm in front of your face and holding the elbow, turn the waist in the opposite direction, maintaining the stretch for fifteen seconds. Perform this exercise in both directions.

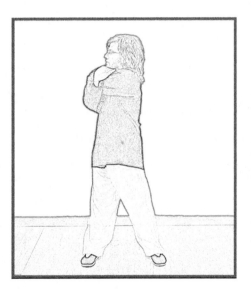 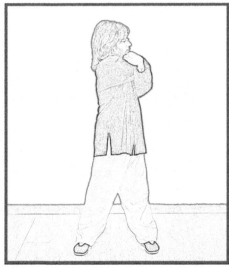

Bringing the palms of your hands together, and interlocking the fingers, perform twenty wrist rotations in each direction..

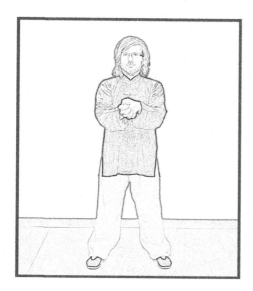 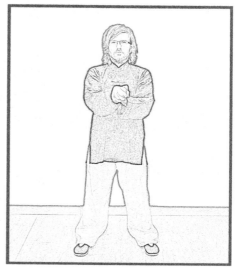

Bringing the backs of your hands together, slowly lower the elbows, gently stretching for twenty seconds.

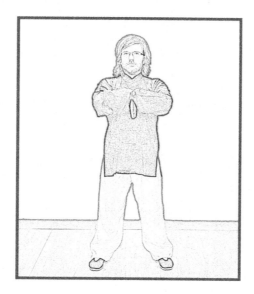

Placing the palm of your hand facing up with the elbow extended, hold the fingers with the other hand and gently stretch the tendons for fifteen seconds. Repeat the exercise with the other arm.

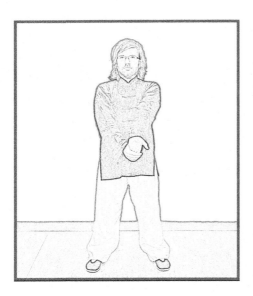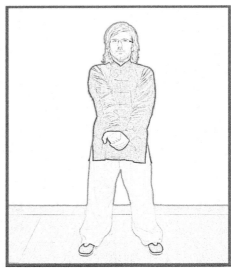

Spreading your legs, make circles with your waist and hips, twelve repetitions in each direction.

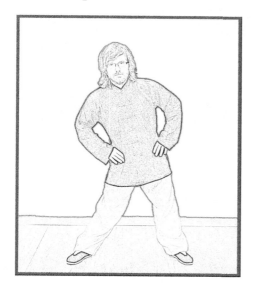 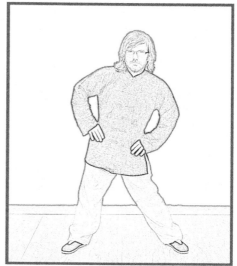

Bringing your feet together again, and resting your hands on the femur, slowly make circles with your knees, twelve times in each direction.

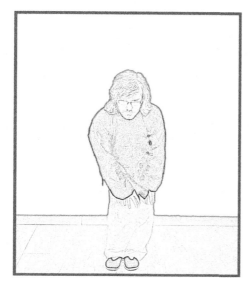 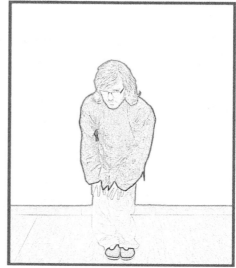

In the same position, bend and straighten your knees. Twelve repetitions.

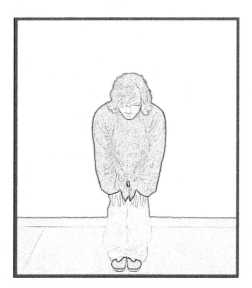 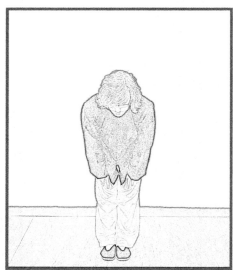

Spreading your legs, bend one knee and straighten the other. Turn your waist in the direction that the bent leg indicates, and direct the toe of the other foot in the same line. Stay in this position for fifteen seconds and repeat with the other leg.

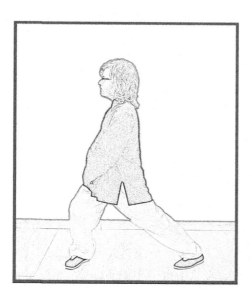 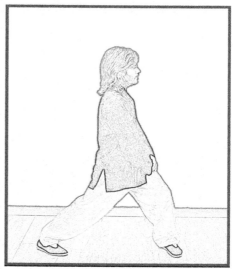

Placing your weight on one leg, lift the heel of the opposite foot and make circles with the ankle, a total of fifteen repetitions. Repeat the exercise with the other leg.

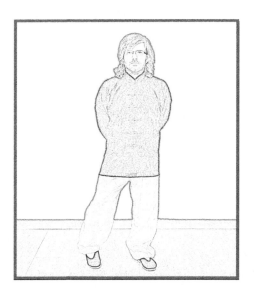
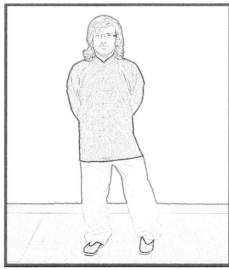

Spreading your legs shoulder-width, stretch one arm up. With the other hand, hold the wrist and gently stretch sideways for fifteen seconds. Repeat with the other arm.

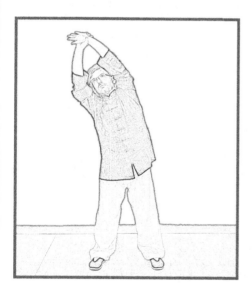 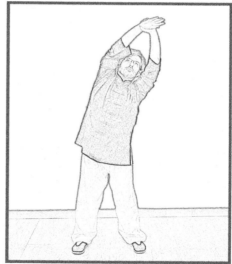

Bringing your feet together, stretch your arms, with the fingers interlocked, upwards. Gently turn your waist keeping your back straight, to one side. Hold this stretching position for fifteen seconds and repeat the exercise on the other side. The waist must turn a maximum of ninety degrees.

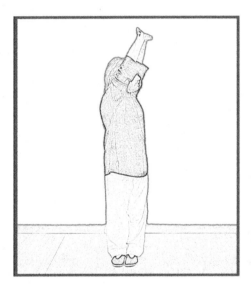 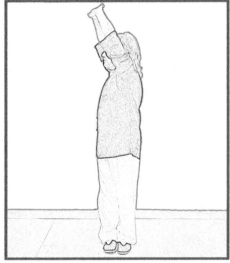

BASIC FOOTWORK

Once the fundamental principles of Tai Chi Chuan have been established, we can build our first tools to work with. Logically, our practice must be focused first of all on consolidating our bow stance. For this, and having in mind all the elements listed in the previous chapter, we will take up the stance on both sides, keeping it steady for a few seconds. Later on, we will be able to prolong the duration of the exercise to perfect our base; the foundation of our study. However, we should avoid overdoing it with the training. Many people, when seeing a Tai Chi practitioner execute a Form or exercise, tend to think that it is light work in which it is not necessary to make any effort. However, the reality is very different. In terms of physical stress, Tai Chi is a demanding discipline that requires technique and progressive learning, adequate to the capacities of the student. We should always advance from less to more, gradually and consistently.

The next stage of the work consists in performing successive steps, both forward and backward, alternating both sides of the stance. To do this, we have to bear in mind two fundamental factors that guarantee our balance and the integrity of the position. First of all, we must remember that every time we move one leg or foot, the body weight must rest on the other limb. We should also have in mind that the forty-five-degree angle that the feet trace must be maintained for the stance to be solid and stable. Therefore, when we want to advance one step towards the next stance, the first thing we have to do is transfer the weight to the back leg. This way, this leg will become *full*, or *Yang*; and the leg in front will be *empty*, or *Yin*. Once the weight is on the back leg, we can modify the angle of the front foot to forty-five degrees, since this is going to be the supporting leg to move forward.

Once we have done this, we can shift our weight to the front leg and advance to a middle stance that will help us maintain balance. Then, we can advance opening the step to the width of the third line and distribute our body weight to fifty percent on each leg, thus adopting, once again, the bow stance. Once we have progressed in our training, we will be able to leave out the middle step and perform the whole process in a much smoother way.

It is important to notice that the geometric harmony of the stance is not decomposed during the successive repetitions. In this sense, we have to bear in mind that the length of the step is not the same when we advance as to when we move backwards. As I've already indicated, in the bow stance the body weight rests on both legs equally, and, as a consequence, the length of the step must be the one that allows the knee of the front leg to stop approximately over the centre of the sole. However, as we move backwards, we place our body weight on the back leg, so the steps must be shorter to keep balance and avoid any type of injury.

It is necessary that you practise these movements, putting special emphasis on correcting the stance, so that you may continue your learning with guarantees of success.

STEPS FORWARD

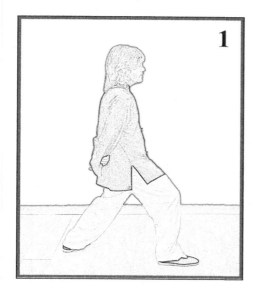 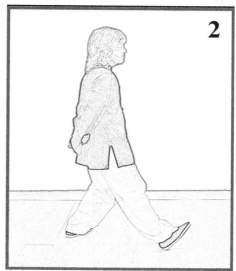

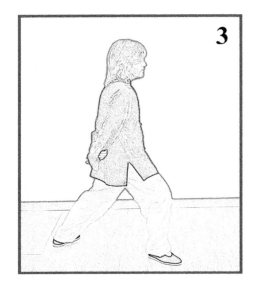

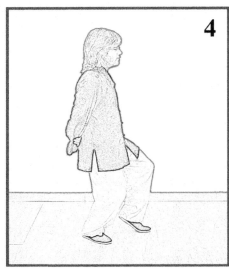

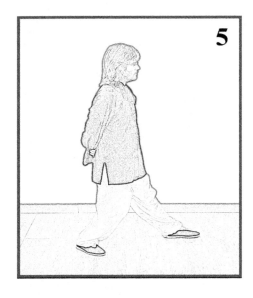

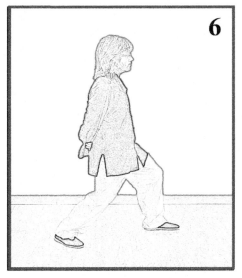

STEPS BACKWARD

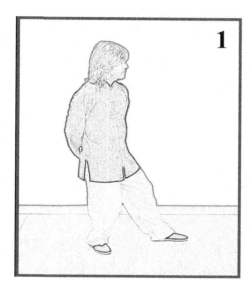

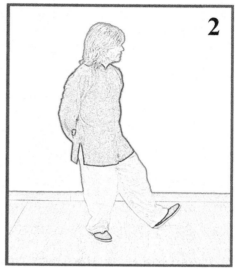

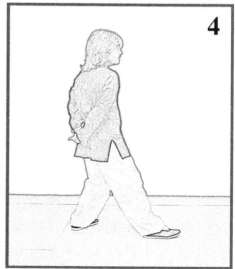

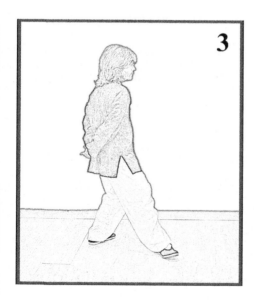

DESCRIPTION OF THE TECHNIQUES

Tai Chi Chuan, like many other traditional Chinese Martial Arts, is very extensive and consists of a great number of techniques. However, and given that this manual means to present the practice of Tai Chi as a tool to improve the general state of health of the student, our work will focus on the reduced number of techniques that allow us to achieve the desired goals in a logical timeframe. Apart from that, many of the techniques that form part of Tai Chi Chuan require more in-depth training and could be harmful to the people to whom this book is directed. Thus, I am going to describe a series of techniques that you should learn little by little, to later add them to the Tai Chi Form with which we will culminate the learning work that we have undertaken in this book.

As is logical, I am not going to get into the explanation of these techniques from a martial point of view, but I will limit myself to demonstrating their execution from a strictly educational point of view. Remember that you should take into account all of the elements described in the section dedicated to the bow stance. In such a way that, even though all the steps and details that make up each technique are numbered one by one, the final execution should be considered one sole movement, correctly carrying out the weight shifts and the waist rotation. For our study, the only exceptions to these rules are the techniques *Beginning posture* and *Hands strum the pipá*.

BEGINNING POSTURE

This technique opens the vast majority of traditional Tai Chi Chuan Forms and is also often used as an exercise in external Chi Kung. For its performance, place your feet to the width of your shoulders and rest your palms on the front part of the legs. Then relax the shoulders and chest as much as possible. In this position, slightly balance forward, at the same time as you begin to raise the relaxed arms to the width and height of the shoulders. Then, start lowering your arms to the waist, palms facing down, and slightly bend your knees, trying to keep your back straight and tuck the pelvis. To correctly learn this apparently simple technique, it is advisable to perform series of eight repetitions.

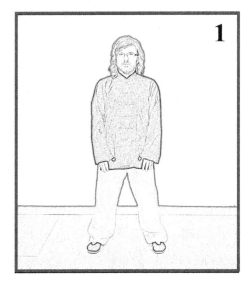

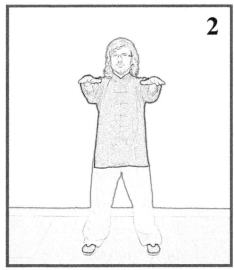

Front view

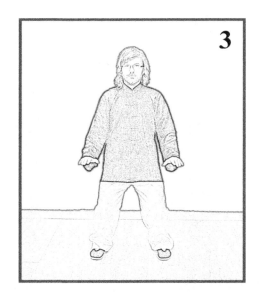

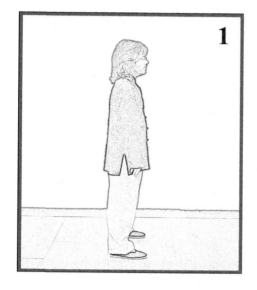

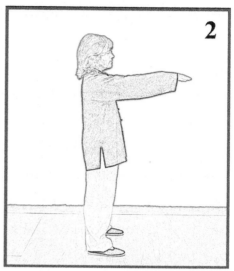

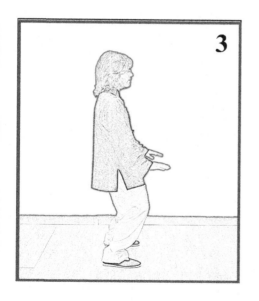

Side view

PARTING WILD HORSE'S MANE

To perform this technique, start from the middle step described in the previous chapter. You can begin on any of the sides interchangeably. For example, if you place your body weight on the left leg to advance to a right leg bow stance, bring your left hand to the height of your right shoulder. Place your right hand, palm facing up, below the navel. The waist has to turn slightly to the left side. In this way, you will be taking up the basic guard stance of Tai Chi Chuan, which we are not going to analyse. Upon opening the bow stance, raise your right arm to the height of your right shoulder, and lower the left one until it is parallel to the head of the left femur.

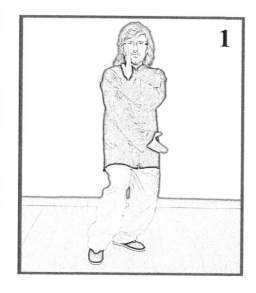

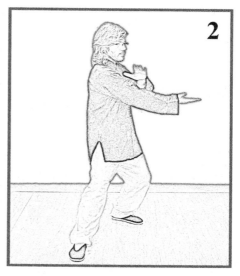

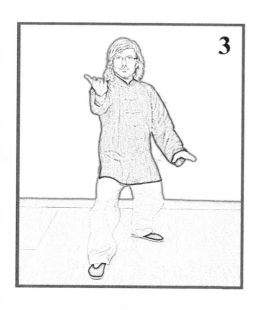

Front view

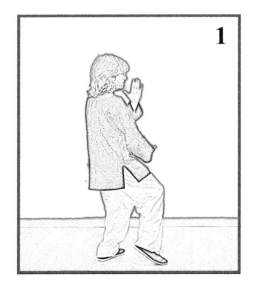

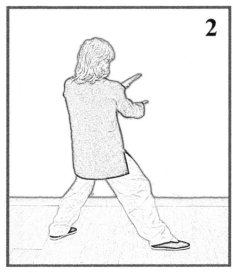

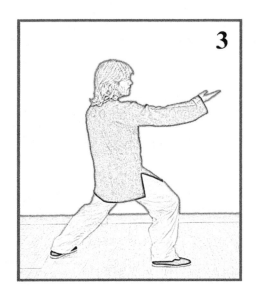

Side view

WHITE CRANE SPREADS ITS WINGS

This technique is executed always on the same side and is exceptionally symmetrical. Place your body weight on the right leg, while your left foot is in front. In this case, we will not perform any weight shift. The waist must be straight. Place your left hand at the height of your right shoulder and the right hand below the navel with the palm facing up. Next, turn the waist forty-five degrees to the left, and, as the waist goes back to its original angle, open the right hand upwards and lower the left one to the head of your left femur. The starting point of this technique often causes confusion among beginners, as it can be similar to the basic guard of Tai Chi. However, these are different stances with different martial applications.

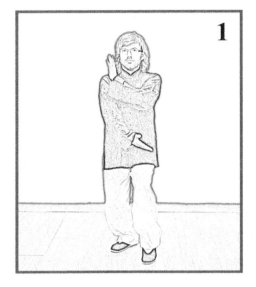

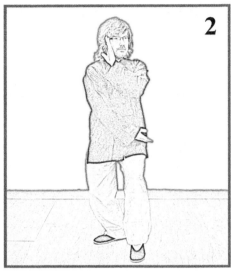

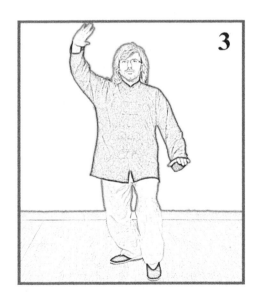

Front view

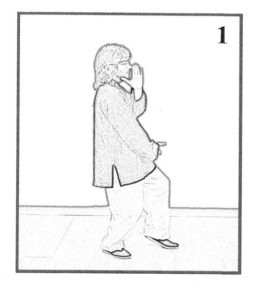

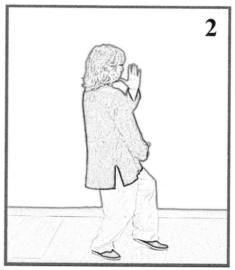

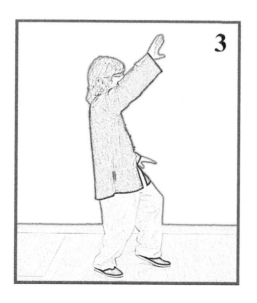

Side view

BRUSH KNEE TWIST STEP

The stance and footwork are the same as in the technique *Parting wild horse's mane*. In this case, from the initial starting point, the right hand, placed at the height of the temple with the palm facing down, advances to a frontal position showing the palm forward, while the left hand performs a sweeping circular movement that ends next to the knee.

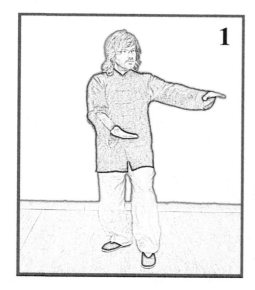

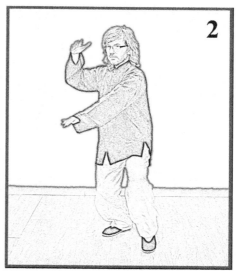

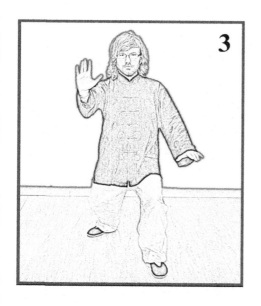

Front view

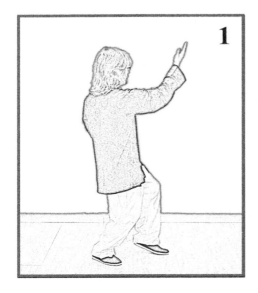

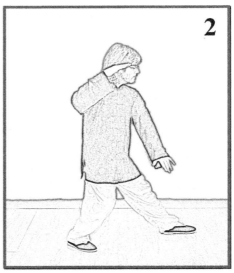

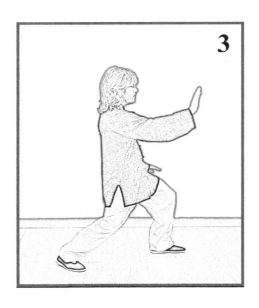

Side view

HAND STRUMS THE PIPÁ

This technique constitutes an exception to the established guidelines regarding the structure of the Tai Chi stance, since the feet are not separated from each other by the distance marked by the third line, but are placed parallelly. Even though we can practise this technique on any of the two sides, I am going to explain it exactly as it appears in the Tai Chi Form that I will describe in the next chapter. Put your weight on the right leg, with the ball of the foot forming a forty-five-degree angle. Place your left foot forward in a straight line with the toe up. Your left arm, almost stretched, is placed in front of the face with the palm in a vertical position, while your right hand must remain at the height of your left elbow, with the palm directed towards it.

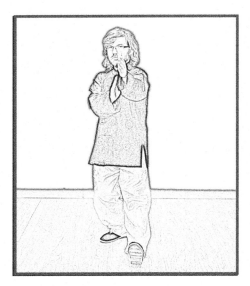

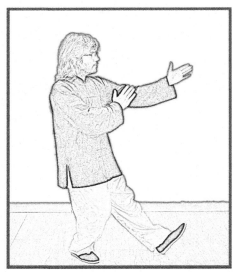

Front view   **Side view**

STEP BACK AND REPULSE THE MONKEY

From the *Hand strums the pipá* position, move the leg that was in front to the back, supporting the foot with the ball at a forty-five-degree angle and the width of the third line. Then, place your weight on the back leg, and correct the angle of the foot in front, directing the toe forward. Make a circular motion with your right hand until the palm is exposed, at the same time as turning your waist, while moving your left hand up, turning the palm upwards, until it rests below the navel. It is very important to have in mind that, even though retreats start from the *Hand strums the pipá* stance, we must respect the third line just as when we are advancing in the bow stance.

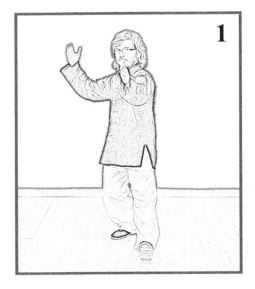

1

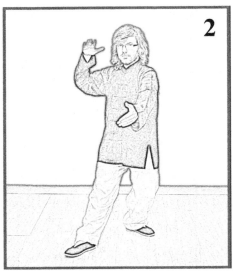

2

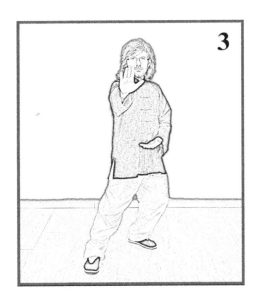

3

Front view

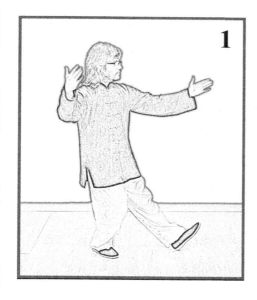

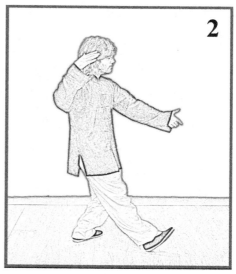

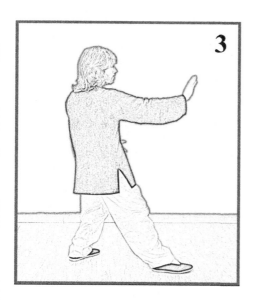

Side view

73

SEQUENCE: WARD OFF, ROLL BACK, PRESS, PUSH

Although these are five different techniques, it is common to learn them in a sequence since they are usually found one after the other in the same order. Starting from the basic guard, with your weight placed on the left leg, open compose the bow stance with your right leg. Raise your right arm to the front with the palm facing inwards, while your left hand remains stable, slightly above the elbow. Turn your waist forty-five degrees to the right: *Ward off*.

Next, turn your palms until reversing their position and, while rotating the waist to a total of ninety degrees to the left, shift your body weight to your left leg: *Roll back*.

Place the outer part of your left palm behind your right wrist, turn the waist to the centre and put the body weight on both legs until you are in a bow stance: *Press*.

Turning both palms downwards, the right hand makes a small circular sweeping move over the right one. Then, put the body weight back on the left leg. Place the arms, almost extended, at the height and width of the shoulders. Presenting the palms of the hands forward, go back to the bow stance with the weight distributed fifty percent on each leg: *Push*.

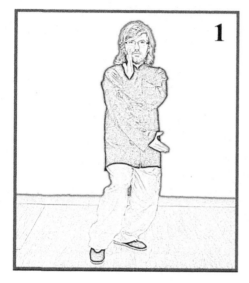

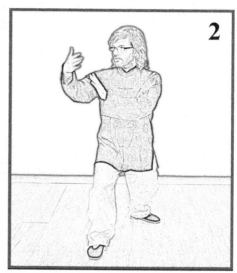

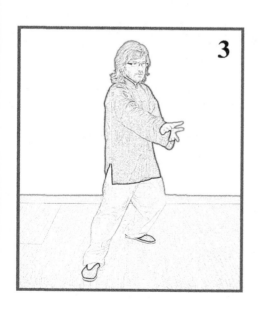

Front view

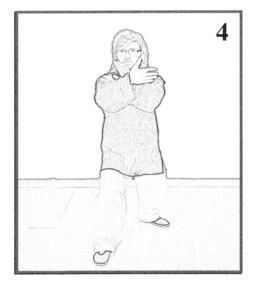

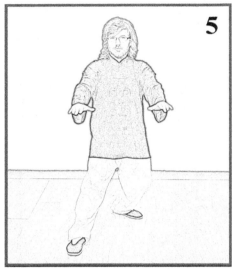

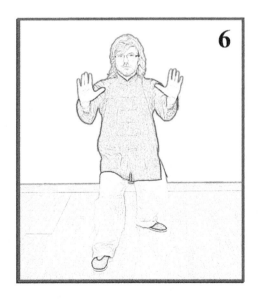

Front view

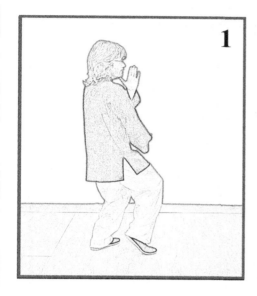

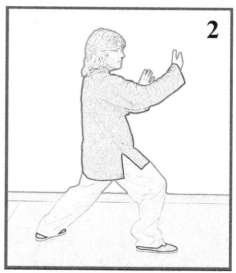

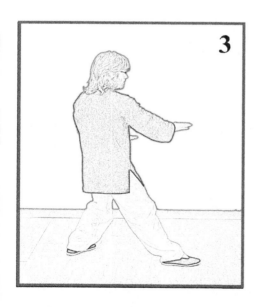

Side view

77

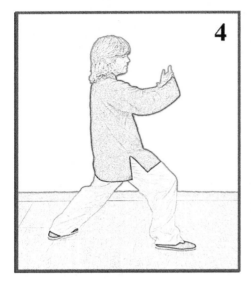

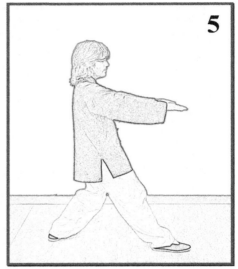

Side view

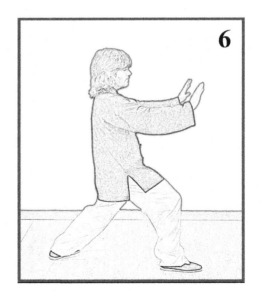

WAVE HANDS LIKE CLOUDS

This technique is characterized by its lateral movement, with the feet parallel to each other. To perform it, you should stand with your feet spread at a distance a bit wider than the width of your shoulders, with your knees semi-bent, and the toes facing forward. The left hand is placed right below the eyes, with the elbow relaxed, lower than the wrist. The right hand rests below the navel with the palm facing up. From this position, turn the waist forty-five degrees to the left. The left hand goes down from the outer side and the right one goes up on the inner side, until reversing their positions, gently turning the palms.

Then, the body weight should be shifted to the left leg to unite the feet bringing the right leg closer. Next, and keeping the feet together, repeat the move turning to the right, slightly pivoting on the ball of your left foot.

The entire sequence must be repeated twice to complete the technique.

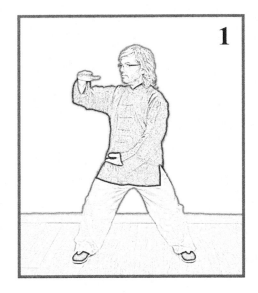

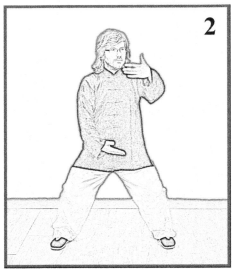

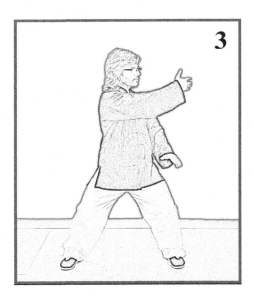

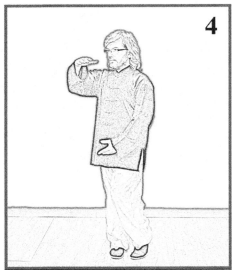

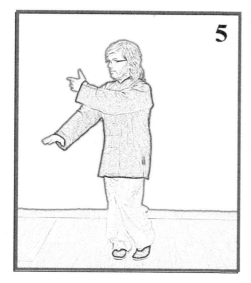 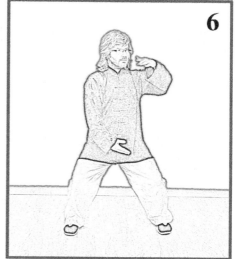

SINGLE WHIP

We will begin the execution of this technique from the bow stance, with the right leg in front, and the arms extended forward almost completely. The palms face the ground.

As we shift our body weight to the left leg and turn the waist, the right arm performs a curvilinear motion until it is at a ninety-degree angle with the left toe. The fingers of the right hand meet in a relaxed way in front of the centre of the palm. At the same time, the left hand turns until the palm is directed inwards, ending up right where the right shoulder is.

Then, we go back to the initial position drawing the left arm parallel to the left leg, we turn the wrist showing the palm of our left hand, and we push gently at the same time as we distribute our body weight to both legs equally.

Later on, when the study of the Tai Chi Form begins, you will perform this technique after *Wave hands like clouds*, one of its most common places. Nevertheless, I advise the decontextualized practice of *Single whip* since it is one of the most difficult executions to learn during the first phases of the work.

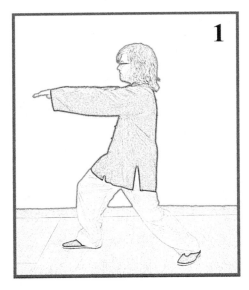 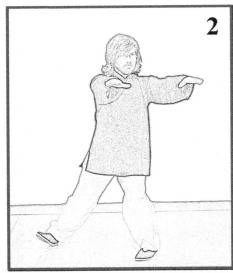

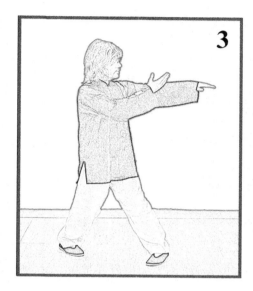

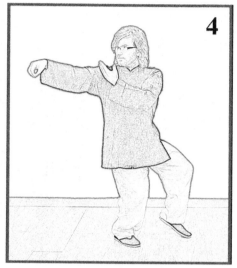

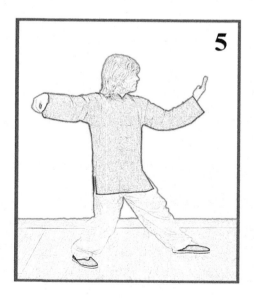

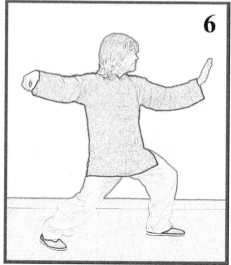

TAI CHI
FORM

"All difficult things have their origin
in that which is easy, and great
things in that which is small."

In the context of traditional Chinese Martial Arts, the Forms contain the technical knowledge of a given style. They are also the vehicle of transmission through the different generations of Masters, and constitute a key element in the qualified study of any martial system: it is not possible to reach deep levels of martial knowledge without studying the Forms. Moreover, the performance of the different Tai Chi Forms in itself is a source of health and serenity, even when said practice is completely disconnected from its martial origin, as it happens in the case of people practising Tai Chi to improve their health, be what they may their objectives on a personal level.

In the case of Yang Style Tai Chi Chuan, there is a great number of empty hand Forms as well as sequences with weapons. Some of these sequences are traditional, while many others have appeared throughout history for the most diverse reasons: from the interest to promote Tai Chi as a cultural element outside the Chinese borders (24-step Form), to the creation of artistic or showy routines directed to sports competition (it is the case for many Forms with weapons). Next, I am going to show you the Form practised by the older people who assist the courses I teach. In this case, it is not a traditional Form, but a simple sequence of techniques created by me for this group of students in particular. All the techniques included in the Form are representative of Yang Tai Chi Chuan. However, I have avoided drawing upon certain stances and movements that could harm untrained people, especially if they are older, since they usually have joint problems, osteoporosis or rheumatisms. We should also bear in mind that the flexibility of the connective tissue diminishes over time, and the tonicity of the muscle mass is lower.

Additionally, this Form is brief and the movements are very basic as it is inscribed in a cross pattern and there is no diagonal technique. In other words, memorizing the entire sequence is relatively easy.

For all these reasons, I think that this Form is adequate for the work we have set as the principal aim of this book: it is short, representative of our martial system, accessible to the vast majority of older people who want to practise Tai Chi and easy to memorize.

First of all, it is necessary to learn the number of repetitions of each technique that we are going to perform, and the direction and orientation of each of them. For this purpose, you should first work on the structure of the Form, taking into account everything explained in the previous chapters. I should point out that, if we want to be loyal to the tradition, the Forms must always be initiated facing the south. This is not arbitrary, and has to do, among other things, with the theory of traditional Chi Kung. However, it is not an issue of decisive importance in the context of our work, and it is normal for every practitioner to adapt to the space available to them.

SCHEME

In this section, I describe the structure of the Tai Chi Form in detail. I do not consider it necessary to add illustrations, since they would be redundant considering that the content of these paragraphs can be observed in the presentation of the complete Form. Thus, the reader can consult the section that contains the Form while studying the text.

To start, you should get into the starting stance: feet together, back straight and relaxed, and hands at the sides. Then slightly bend the knees, placing your weight on your right leg. Lifting the left heel, separate the left foot from the right one until it stops at the width of the shoulders. Rest the left sole on the ground again and place your weight back on both legs at the same time, straightening, then, the knees.

At first, we have to redirect our position towards the left. To do this, it is necessary to shift our body weight to the left leg. Next, pivot on the right heel until placing your foot at a forty-five-degree angle to the left, at the same time as turning the waist in the same direction.

From there, form the bow stance by advancing your left leg.

The next step consists in repeating the same stance, but to the right; for which we must modify the direction of the technique by one hundred and eighty degrees. To achieve this, pivot on your left heel, and take up the bow stance with the right leg forward.

Next, shift the body weight to your left leg and turn your right heel forty-five degrees to the left. Then shifting your weight to the right leg, make three advances in the bow stance, thus recovering the direction the Form started in.

In continuation, slightly shorten the length of the stance by stepping forward with your right foot and execute the stance *Hand strums the pipá*.

From this position, we will make two consecutive steps back.

Placing the body weight on your right leg, adopt the *White crane spreads its wings* stance. From there, take three steps forward again in the bow stance. At this point of the Form, we have to turn to our right again. Therefore, after shifting your weight to the right leg, pivot on your left heel forty-five degrees to the right to correct the direction, and take up the bow stance.

After that, take the lateral steps corresponding to the technique *Wave hands like clouds* and, as previously described, take up the bow stance to the left on which the *Single whip* technique is executed.

To finish, shift the weight to your right leg again and pivot on your left heel towards the frontal position, thus recovering the original direction in which we have started the scheme. Next, shift the weight back to the left leg, and place the right foot at the width of the shoulders; in other words, reproduce the position of the opening in reverse.

Then put the weight back on your right leg, and bring both feet together. Finally, straighten your knees and close the position.

It is essential to learn and dominate this scheme to be able to perform the Tai Chi Form correctly. Once you are comfortable with the stances and steps, you will be able to start training the complete Form, as presented in continuation.

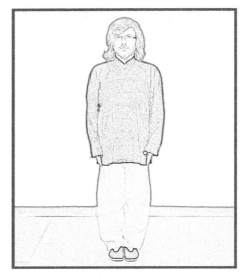 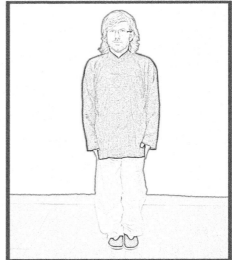

Preparation

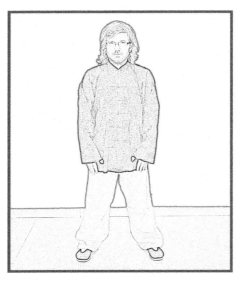 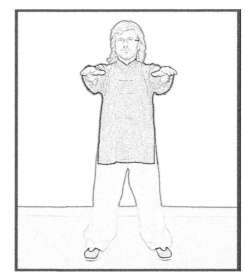

Beggining posture

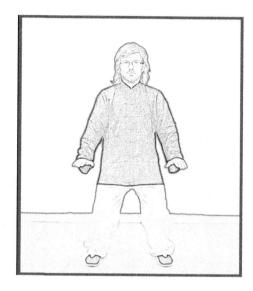
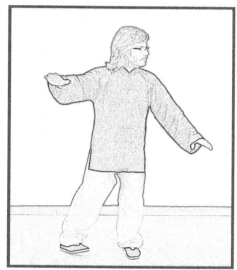
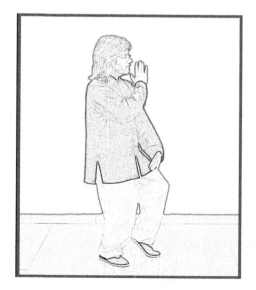
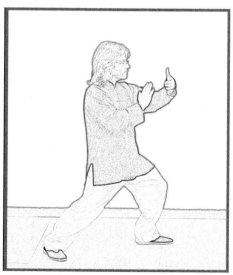

Ward Off

91

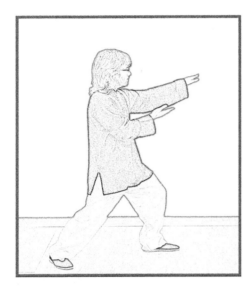

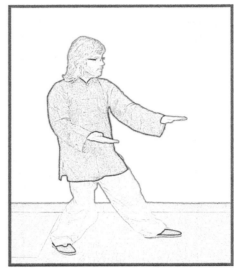

Roll back

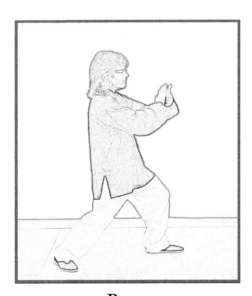

Press

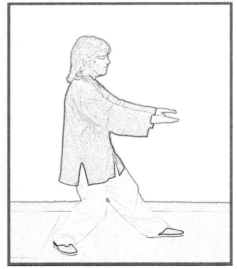

92

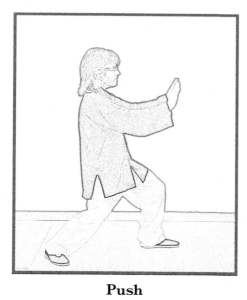

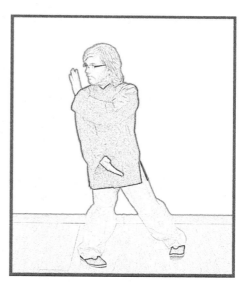

Push

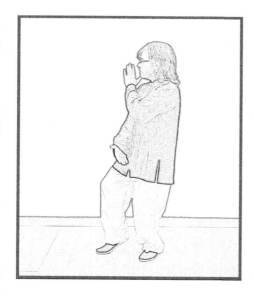

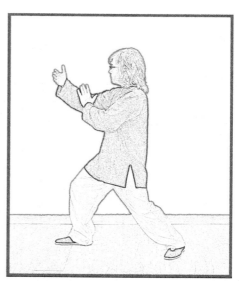

Ward off

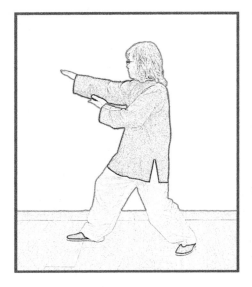

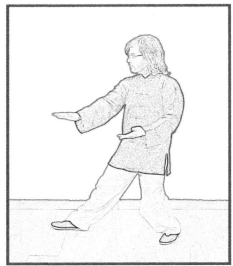

Roll back

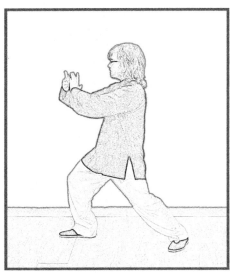

Press

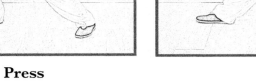

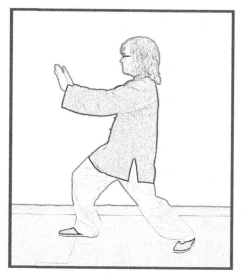

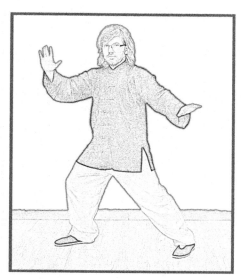

Push

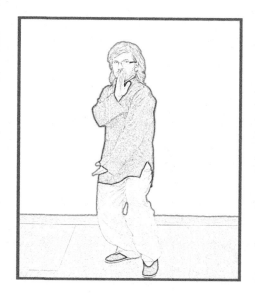

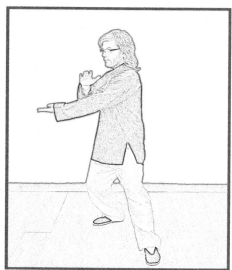

Parting wild horse´s mane

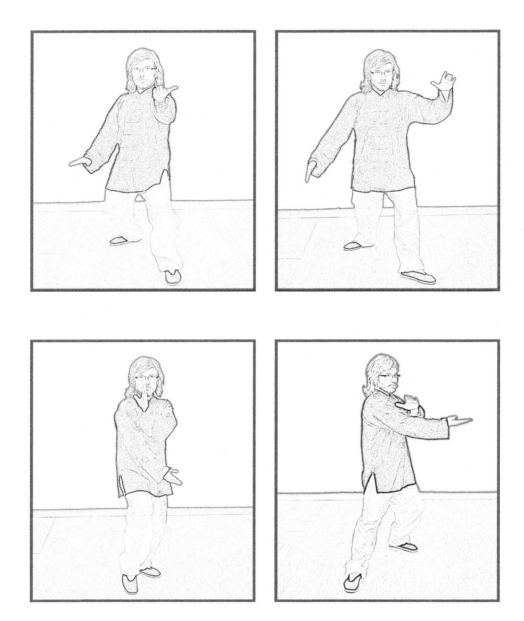

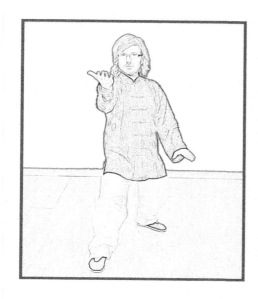
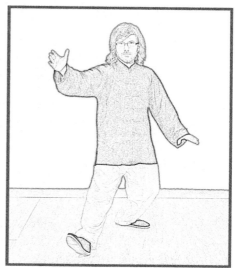

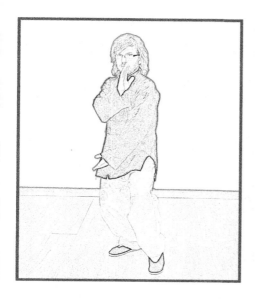
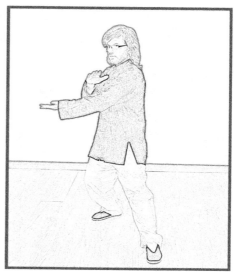

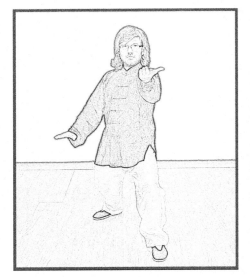

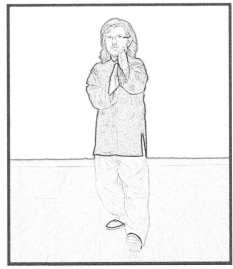

Hand strums the pipá

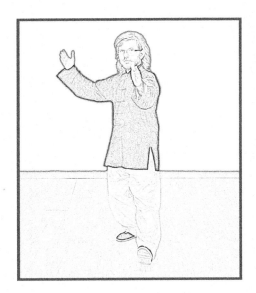

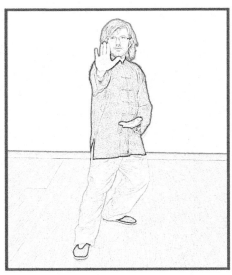

Step back and repulse the monkey

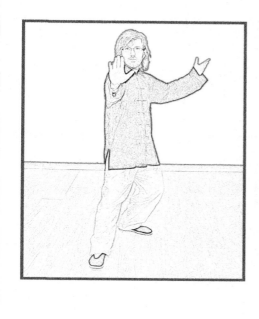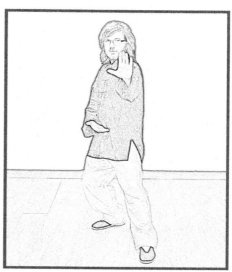

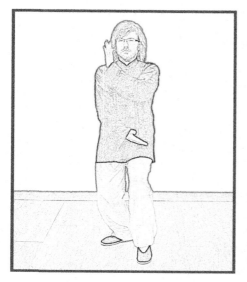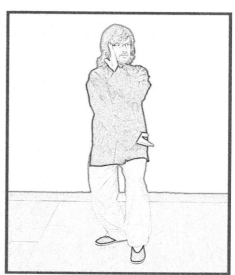

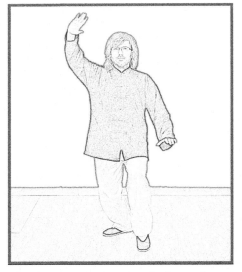
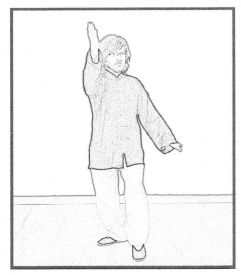

White crane spreads its wings

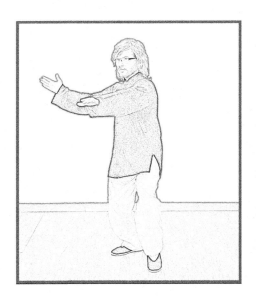
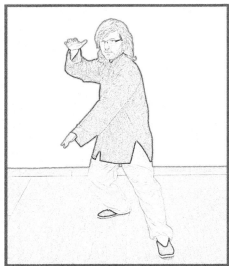

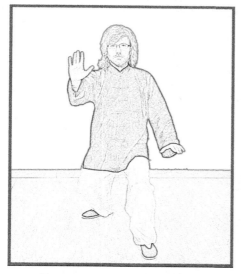 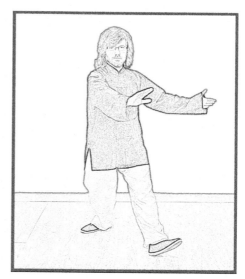

Brush knee twist step

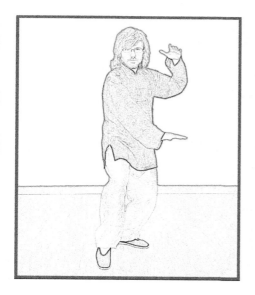 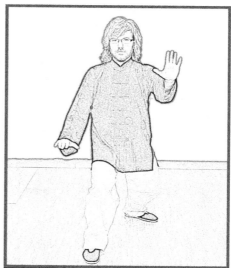

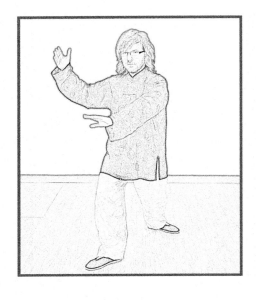 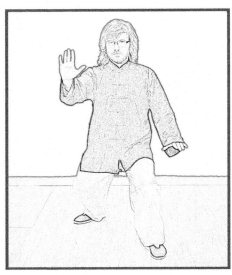

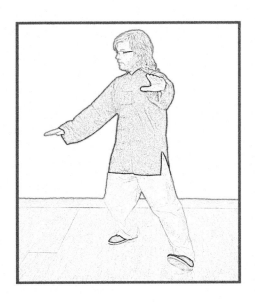 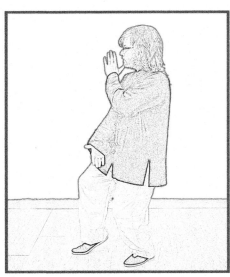

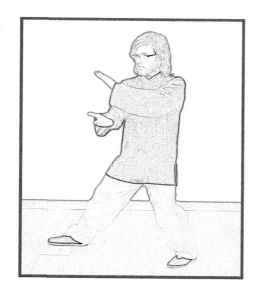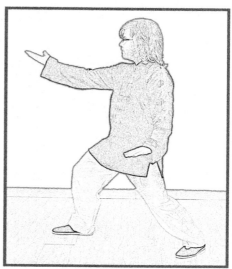

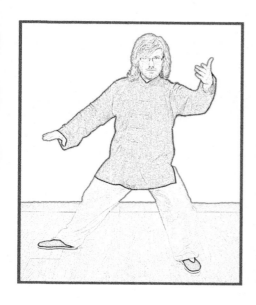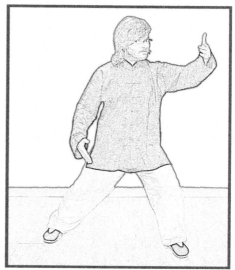

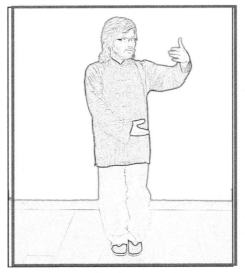 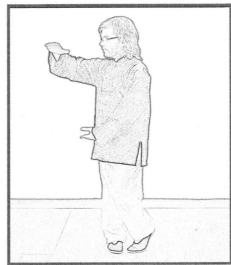

Wave hands like clouds

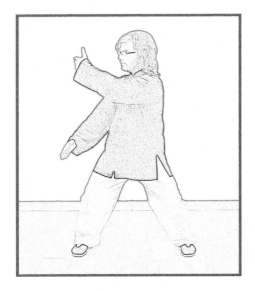 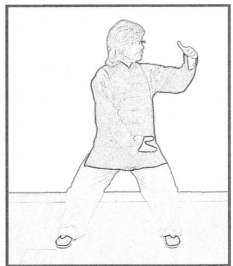

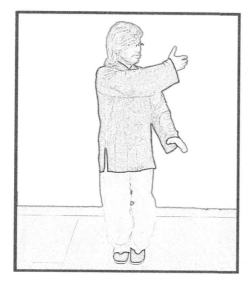

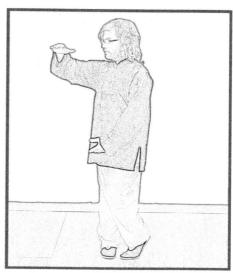

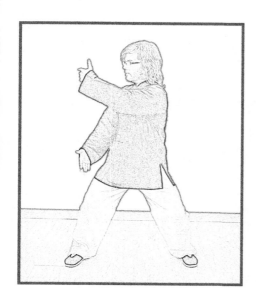

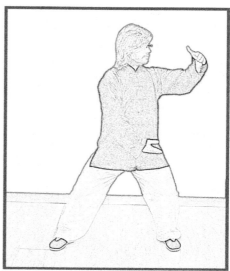

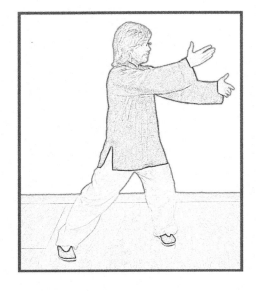
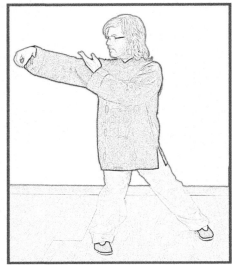

Single whip

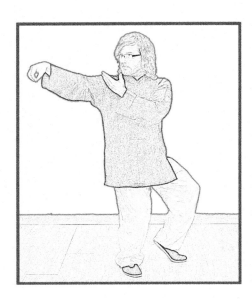
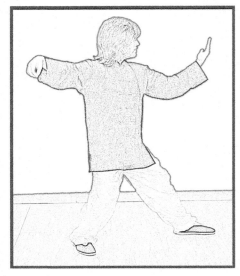

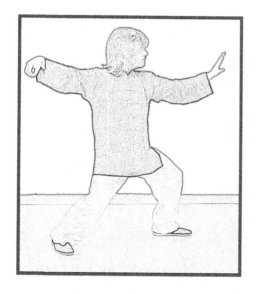
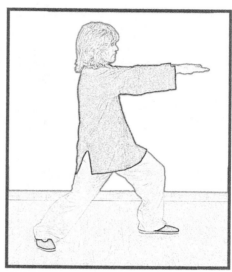

Push

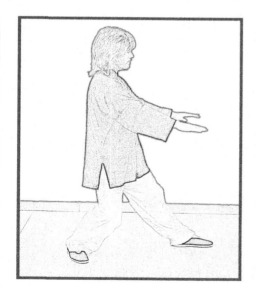
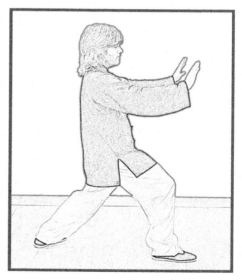

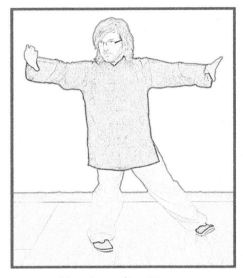
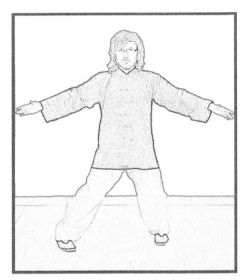

Closing the Form

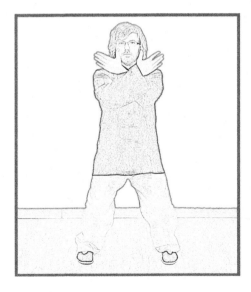
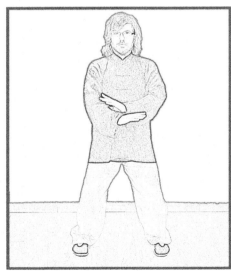

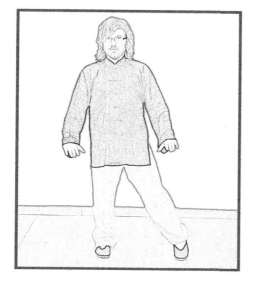 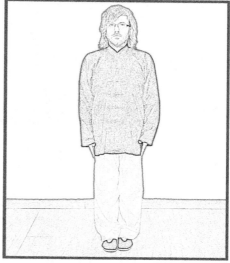

CONCLUSION

"In the pursuit of knowledge, every day something is added. In the practice of the Tao, every day something is dropped."

This is a simple and light book, which renounces developing a complete and systematic analysis of Tai Chi Chuan in favour of accessibility and utility. Even though it is evident that many issues have been left incomplete in their presentation and further explanation, I am confident that I have achieved the main aim that has motivated me to write this manual: to present a comprehensible, useful and accessible tool that will allow older people who wish so to come closer to the study of Tai Chi.

Maybe in a future book, there will be a chance to delve into the various facets that compose the profound knowledge of the Art of Tai Chi Chuan.

In any case, I consider that this book puts at your disposal a great deal of elements of work that, without a doubt, will allow you to successfully initiate into the study of Tai Chi Chuan and, as a consequence of that, work daily to improve your health and grow from a perspective rooted in our ancestral tradition.

Each of the techniques presented here, though they may seem simple at first, have been distilled through generations. Masters and Disciples are the links that forge the millenary chain of tradition, meticulously taking care of the essence of Tai Chi so that it remains unaltered.

It is, thus, a work that must be approached with rigour and respect: Martial Arts always give back to us more than what we have invested in their learning and development. All progress is always a direct consequence of effort. Tenacity, patience and willpower are our most loyal allies on the path of learning.

The following QR code offers access to a video that presents the complete Tai Chi Form, with the purpose of complementing the content of this book.

About the auhtor:

Juan Antonio de Blas was trained at the Chinese Martial Arts School of Grandmaster Pedro Rico, one of the most prominent Sifus in Europe; expert in Kung Fu Choy Li Fut and Yang Tai Chi Chuan, and main representative in Europe of the Plum Blossom International Federation, chaired by Grandmaster Doc Fai Wong.

After participating in national and European championships, where he won first awards in different categories of Kung Fu Choy Li Fut and Yang Tai Chi Chuan, Juan Antonio de Blas now focuses his activity on teaching.

Over the years, he has been giving courses and seminars of Tai Chi Chuan, Kung Fu and Chi Kung for both private and public entities, thus contributing in the promotion and conservation of these traditional disciplines.

In close collaboration with the Zaragoza City Council (Spain), Juan Antonio de Blas has taught Tai Chi Chuan and Chi Kung to more than five hundred students each academic term in the last fifteen years.

This informative work is simultaneously complemented by the publication of articles, and the cycle of conferences Martial Arts and Health, which was offered in collaboration with the government of Aragón and the Zaragoza City Council. He is also the author of the books *Tai Chi sword: Yang style 32 step Form* and *Kung Fu Choy Li Fut - Wooden dummy 36 step Form*.

In order to adapt the traditional performance of Tai Chi, Kung Fu and Chi Kung to the specific needs of different collectives Juan Antonio de Blas sporadically also provides specific courses intended for companies and organizations of diverse natures. In this regard, particular mention may also be made of his work with entities like ASATRA (Aragonese Association for Anxiety Disorder) or CLECE S.A. that provides telecare services for elderly people. Since 2012, he has taught in his own tradional school, Dan Tian, in Zaragoza, Spain.

Printed in Great Britain
by Amazon

37618856R00066